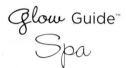

Glow Guide™
Spa

Glow Guide™
Spa

**Simple Steps for
Health and Well-Being**

By Andrea McCloud

Illustrations by
Karen Greenberg

CHRONICLE BOOKS
SAN FRANCISCO

Library of Congress Cataloging-in-Publication Data:

McCloud, Andrea.

Spa : simple steps for health and well-being / by Andrea McCloud ;
illustrations by Karen Greenberg.
p. cm. — (Glow guide)
ISBN 0-8118-4097-2 (pbk.)
1. Relaxation. 2. Detoxification (Health) 3. Herbal cosmetics.
4. Health resorts. I. Title. II. Series.
RA785.M386 2004
613—dc21
2003003782

Manufactured in China

Designed by Greenberg Kingsley/NYC

Distributed in Canada by Raincoast Books
9050 Shaughnessy Street
Vancouver, British Columbia V6P 6E5

10 9 8 7 6 5 4 3 2 1

Chronicle Books LLC
85 Second Street
San Francisco, California 94105

www.chroniclebooks.com

Life is one, big, beautiful spa.

Indulge.

Dedication

To all of the people out there who have
never indulged in a massage, facial,
body treatment, manicure, pedicure,
or something of that nature — it's time.

Acknowledgments

A huge thanks to friends and family for enduring the
Glow Guide: Spa *clinical trials. Additional thanks
to all of the spa technicians I badgered with phone
calls and "office" visits. Special thanks to my editor,
Mikyla Bruder, for her guidance (and impeccable
taste), and to the kids at Chronicle Books for their
hard work and dedication. A final and titanic thank
you to my former boss and Chronicle Books' associate
publisher, Christine Carswell, for opening the floodgates.*

Contents

Spa treatments are for more than just simple rest and relaxation. The recipes in this book can do everything from banish the occasional breakout to wake up dry, tired hair. Here's a list of quick cures for what might ail you.

Quick Fixes

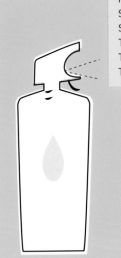

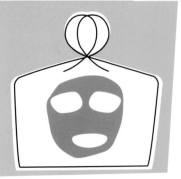

Introduction

Glow is a state of being, a delicate blend of good mental and physical health, personal happiness, self-understanding, and self-confidence. You can't apply it, you can't wear it, and you can't special-order it; glow comes from within. It's an inner radiance that is realized by taking care of yourself and being good to yourself. It's you at your best.

Glow isn't something you approach willy-nilly. Personal radiance is not easy, and it doesn't happen spontaneously—achieving and maintaining it takes time and effort. It's a commitment you make to yourself, a commitment you make to your mind, body, and soul. Cultivating glow is a conscious choice to nurture and pamper yourself, your whole self, not once a month, not once a week, but *every day*.

For many of us, the idea of pampering ourselves seems a bit self-indulgent, perhaps even a trifle gratuitous. It's something you do on special occasions, or *maybe* after a particularly difficult week. But every day? No way. Who's got time for that?

You do! Taking time out for yourself—treating yourself, indulging yourself—is a vital part of your health and happiness, even (I daresay), your sanity. We all want and need an occasional escape, even if it's just a momentary one, from the chaos and intensity of the daily grind. Day after day, week after week, we're pulled this way, pushed that way, stressed, anxious, exhausted, never looking up for a moment to see just how much our mind, body, and soul desperately need attention, never slowing down long enough to notice just how badly we've been treating ourselves. It's time to slow down. It's time to pamper.

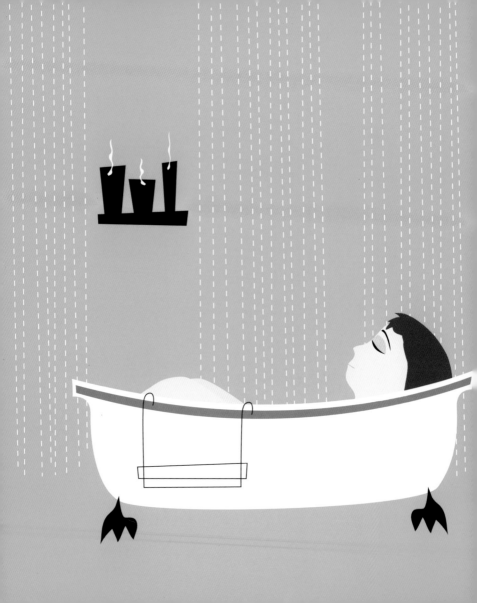

Spotlight the spa. A centuries-old wellness tradition, the spa goes beyond facials and salt scrubs. Sure, looking good is part of it, but more than that the spa is about feeling good. And not sometimes—all the time. This book approaches the spa as a mind-set. The idea being that if you've got the right attitude and are equipped with the right tools, you can achieve a true spa experience no matter where you are. No more once-a-year appointment at some extravagant resort. You can plop down at the spa in your very own bathroom, at your desk, even in your car on the way to work. It's really that simple.

Packed with facial masks, massages, hair treatments, breathing exercises, yoga, meditation, and various other means to achieving mind-body-soul bliss, *Glow Guide: Spa* makes it easy for you to indulge in a little spa treatment every day. It is divided into five chapters: Morning Energizers, Daytime Detoxifiers, Afternoon Revitalizers, Evening Relaxers, and Overnight Rejuvenators; the treatments in each chapter correspond with what you might need—energy, detoxification, revitalization, relaxation, rejuvenation— throughout the day. Stop squandering your precious time on stress and anxiety and instead use it to treat yourself. You'll look better, but most importantly, you'll feel better. In fact, you'll feel great! You'll see.

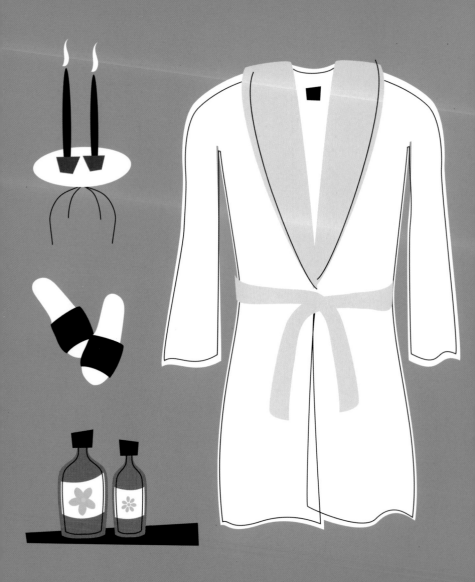

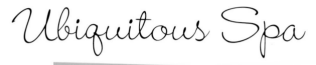

Ubiquitous Spa

Setting the Mood

Yes, the spa is everywhere if you're carrying the right tools. Here are a few suggestions for creating the spa atmosphere wherever you go.

Home Spa

Lighting: Think ambience. Turn down the lights; if possible, use only candlelight. Its soft glimmer will soothe and relax you.

Scent: Essential oils are indeed essential to your home spa. Check out the selection at your local health-food store and pick out your favorites. Aromatherapy candles and incense are another option.

Sound: Listening to silence is, of course, a wonderful way to release stress and tension. But when you're in the mood, quiet, moody music or the sounds of nature will also soothe your soul.

Nature: Bring the outside in with a bouquet of freshly cut flowers. Or, for a bit of simple elegance, float a single blossom in a bowl of water.

Solitude: Time alone is the very essence of spa and should be your biggest priority. Tell your friends and family you are out of commission for the evening. Don't feel guilty about taking the night (or an entire afternoon) to yourself—you deserve it.

Fun stuff: When creating your home spa, you absolutely must treat yourself to the appropriate spa accoutrements: fluffy cotton towels, terry-cloth robe, hair turban, slippers, pumice stone, sea sponge, and natural-bristle brush.

Take the Spa with You

Car Spa

Mellow music

Positive attitude

Moisturizer

A cup holder
full of flora

Sweet almond oil

Cotton gloves

Bottle of water

Exercise gear

Office Spa

Candle

Mini essential-oil set

Tea set and a
selection of tasty teas

Bowl of marbles
(or a golf ball)

Fresh fruit

A cucumber

Facial mist

A plant or freshly
cut flowers

Pair of sneakers

Bottle of water

Traveling Spa

Pack of sugar

Honey

A few bags of your
favorite tea

Portable essential-oil set

Moisturizer

Facial mist

Eye mask

Golf ball

Bottle of water

Slippers

Hair turban

Pillow mist

Bathrobe

Elements of Glow

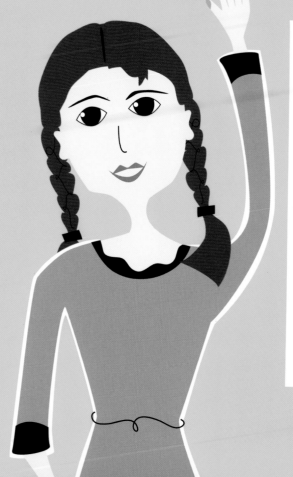

Eat well.

Sleep.

Drink lots of water.

Exercise, exercise, exercise!

Meditate.

Tend to your hair, skin, and nails.

Breathe consciously.

Laugh often.

Pamper yourself.

Don't worry.

Don't judge.

Slow down.

Pay attention.

Be kind.

CHAPTER ONE

Morning Energizers

A quiet time of awakening and revival, the morning is the perfect opportunity for a little spa treatment to rouse a still-sleepy mind, body, and soul. Tomorrow get up a few minutes early and indulge. The treatments in this chapter were chosen specifically for their energizing qualities. Wake up with an early-morning soak, bask in the silence of a sunrise meditation, or pamper yourself with a prework facial mask. If you have an hour or even just five minutes, there's something in here for you.

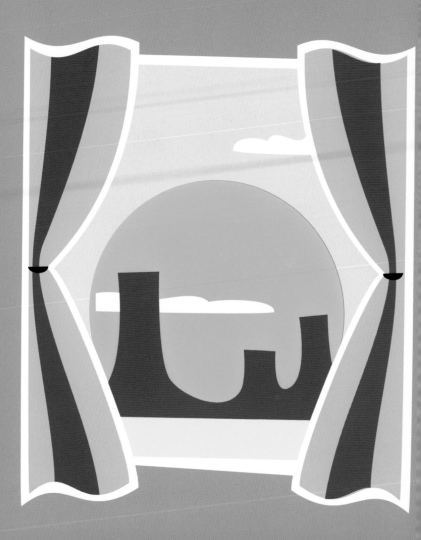

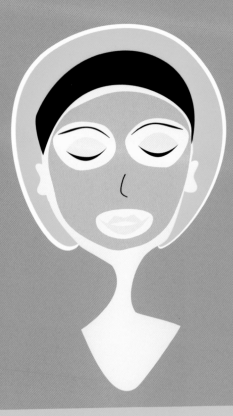

Glow-How

Throwing on a mask before the shower is an easy way to fit a facial treatment into a busy schedule. If you don't have time to mix something together, you can always use a plain yogurt mask—it's a simple but wonderful skin-softening cleanser that's high in vitamins, and smooths skin texture.

Your skin will feast on this ever-so-simple mask of rolled oats, egg, and honey. Rich in vitamins, old-fashioned oatmeal is a mild and gentle cleanser that also nourishes the skin—the perfect morning meal for your face. Bon appétit! (While you're at it, make an extra bowl of oats for breakfast. Eating oatmeal is also good for your complexion. It is loaded with vitamin B, which promotes skin-cell growth, and is packed with fiber, which eliminates toxins, helping to keep skin pimple-free.)

Food for Your Face

What You'll Need

Pot

1 cup water

½ cup oatmeal (slow-cooking rolled oats, not that instant stuff)

Bowl

1 egg

2 teaspoons honey

* Heat the water. When it comes to a boil, add the oatmeal. Reduce heat to medium and cook for about eight minutes, give or take a minute. Remove from the heat and wait five to ten minutes for the oatmeal to cool down.

* In a bowl, mix the egg, honey, and oatmeal together until they form a paste.

* Starting at your neck and working up to your forehead, gently apply the mask, moving your fingers in a continuous circular motion. Make sure to avoid the eye area.

* Leave the mask on for ten minutes. Take this time to do a yoga pose or two, read the paper, or just sit and breathe.

* Shower. Before you rinse off the mask, spend a moment soaking in the steam and gently massaging your face and neck. This will help exfoliate any buildup of dead skin cells.

* Rinse your face and enjoy the rest of your morning ablutions.

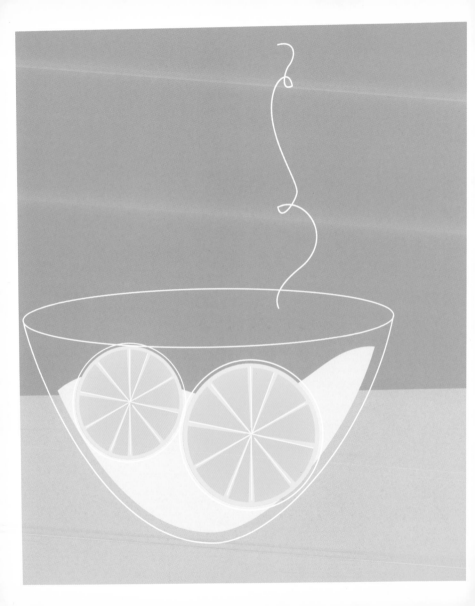

Committing to a ritualistic once-a-week facial steam can work wonders on your complexion. Steaming not only increases circulation in the face, it also helps clean the skin from the inside out, opening the pores and allowing the face to sweat out toxins and impurities. And by throwing a little lemon into the mix, you'll get a zap of energy from the citrus scent.

Citrus Steam

* Put the water on the stove so it can start heating up.

* Wash your face, and then wash it again. The first washing removes surface dirt; the second round will get the stubborn stuff that's hiding a little deeper.

* When the water has come to a boil, squeeze both lemon halves into the pot and then drop them into the water. Cover and let sit for a minute.

* Put the pot on a table and sit down in front of it. Make sure you're comfortable; you'll be sitting in this position for ten to fifteen minutes.

* Drape the towel over your head and put your face about eight to ten inches above the pot. Make sure the towel extends below the rim of the pot; you don't want to lose any of that precious steam.

* Relax and savor your steam. Breathe deeply.

* When your ten minutes are up, rinse with warm water, cleaning out the pores, and then splash your face with a blast of cold water to close them. This is very important, so don't skip this step!

* Steaming can remove a lot of the natural oils from the face, so before you head out the door, be sure to moisturize.

What You'll Need:
___

Large pot

2 quarts of water

1 lemon, cut in half

Towel

Glow-How
___

Don't worry if you have a minor breakout a day or two after steaming; the impurities built up in the skin are simply being flushed out. And this is a good thing. As you continue to steam, the break-outs will subside and your skin will look absolutely radiant. Trust me.

Hot lemon water isn't just for facial steams; it's also good to drink. While its tart taste and citrus scent perk you up, the drink also flushes out the liver, kidneys, and colon and revs up the bowels. So give your system the advantage of a fresh, clean start, and begin your day with a steaming cup of lemon water.

Lemon-Water Elixir

* Heat the water and pour it into the mug.

* Squeeze the lemon into the water.

* Sip, enjoying the tart and tangy taste as the lemon water flushes out your system.

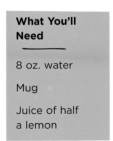

What You'll Need

8 oz. water

Mug

Juice of half a lemon

Glow-How

If possible (and I realize this is asking a lot), try replacing your morning coffee ritual with the much healthier lemon-water ritual. While caffeine does give you that nice early-morning jolt, it also taxes your liver and drains your body of valuable minerals—not a good way to start the day.

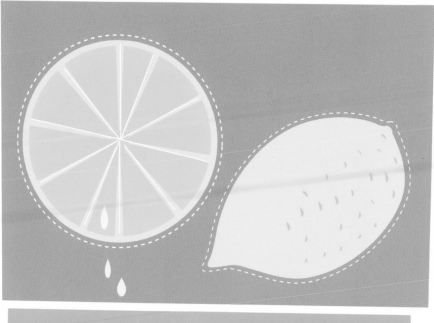

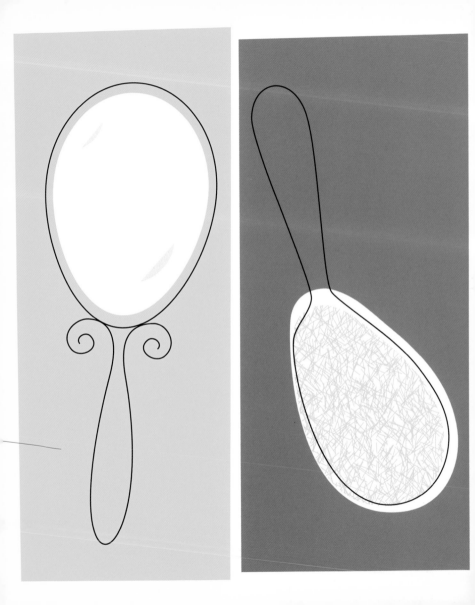

Dry brushing is a morning must. Beyond simple exfoliation, it also increases circulation, helps break down fatty deposits and reduce cellulite (hurrah! back flip, back flip), and aids in the elimination of toxins from your body by stimulating the lymph system. All you need is a natural-bristle body brush and five minutes.

Body Buff

* As you might have guessed, dry brushing is done dry—i.e. no water, soap, lotion, or oils—so do the treatment before you shower. (This will also allow you to rinse off all of the exfoliated skin cells once you've finished brushing.)

* When you're dry brushing, your strokes should always move toward your heart. Begin at your feet and in smooth, sweeping motions work your way up your legs. From your hands, move up your arms; then down your neck, back, and chest; and complete the treatment with a circular motion at the abdomen.

* Take it easy and don't overdo it. Your skin is most likely not used to this type of workout. Over time you can begin to brush with a bit more vigor, but never to the point of discomfort—remember, this is supposed to be an enjoyable experience.

* Once your body is buffed, take a shower or bath, pat yourself dry, and revel in your skin's new glow.

Glow-How

As you can imagine, your brush will need a good cleaning about once a week. Simply wash it with a bit of soap and water and then let it air-dry before you use it again.

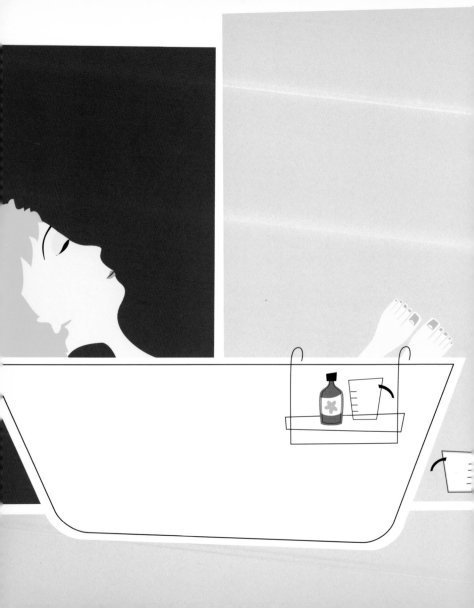

Baths are not just for the evening. Mix it up a little bit; tomorrow, skip the shower and indulge in an early-morning soak. It is a great way to wake up your mind, body, and soul, especially if you add a stimulating essential oil like peppermint, sage, or eucalyptus. For an even bigger energy boost, turn the water temperature down a few degrees. The slight chill (it's only slight, so stop scrunching your nose) will revitalize and invigorate you.

Bathing Bliss

* Draw a bath. Try to keep the temperature slightly below what you're used to—the water should be lukewarm, not hot.

* Add the baking soda and Epsom salts to the running water.

* Add the eucalyptus essential oil.

* Step into the tub, sit back, and relax. Take a deep breath. Hold it for a moment and then release. Feel your mind, body, and soul slowly come alive.

* Enjoy this peaceful time alone. It may be all you get today.

What You'll Need

1 cup
baking soda

1 cup
Epsom salts

6 drops
eucalyptus
essential oil

Glow-How

If you have dry hair, here's an easy addition to your bath-time ritual that will leave your tresses nourished and shiny. Simply combine an entire mango and two tablespoons of honey, massage the mixture into your wet hair, and when you've finished lounging in the tub, rinse.

If a morning bath is too unorthodox for you, the shower can also serve as effective hydrotherapy. Instead of your habitual quick rinse, turn your morning shower into an awakening ritual by adding a splash of sparkling water mixed with jasmine oil. Not only will it stimulate your mind and soften your skin, the sweet scent of jasmine will linger with you all day long.

Jasmine Shower

* Combine the sparkling water and jasmine oil in a bowl and set it inside the shower.

* Ease into the shower. Don't think about the day to come; just be present with yourself and your breath. Breathe consciously and rhythmically.

* Wash as you normally would. Slow down and take your time. Be gentle with yourself and focus on what you're doing.

* When you've finished washing, sponge the sparkling water and jasmine oil over your body, starting at your neck and working your way down to your feet.

* Rinse with a blast of cold water to increase your energy and circulation and to close your pores.

* *Gently* pat yourself dry—you don't want to rub off any of that precious oil—with a fluffy terry-cloth towel.

What You'll Need

3 cups
sparkling water

4 drops
jasmine oil

Bowl

Sea sponge

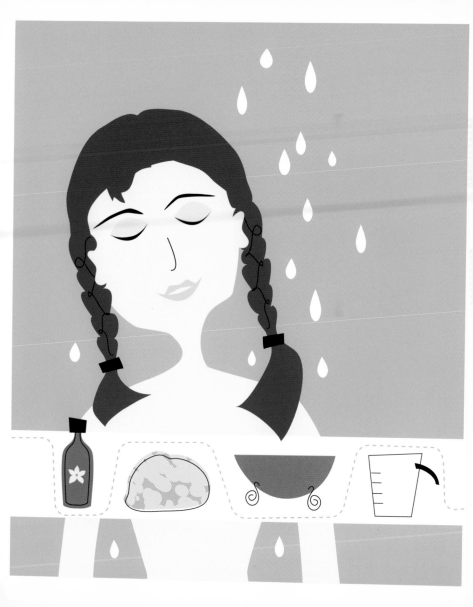

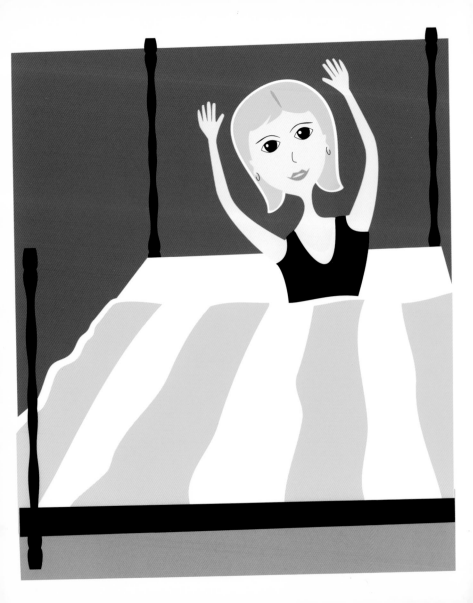

After a solid night's sleep, there is nothing like a good stretch to wake a groggy mind and body. Stretching will not only relieve tense and tight muscles, it will also boost your circulation, upping your energy. And the best part: you don't even need to get out of bed. Love that.

S-t-r-e-t-c-h!

* Throw the sheets to the side and lie on your back. Take a deep breath in through your nose. Feel your chest rise and fall.

* Stretch your arms over your head. Pretend someone has grabbed your hands and feet and is pulling in opposite directions. Stretch your hands up as far as you can and extend your torso. Feel your body lengthening.

* Keep your arms over your head and sit up slowly. Bend forward at the waist and try to grab your toes. Hold this forward bend for twenty seconds.

* Slowly lift up and lie on your back again. Bring your knees to your chest and wrap your arms around your knees, grabbing opposite forearms, or elbows if you can. Put your chin to your chest. Hold for twenty seconds.

* Extend your arms out from your shoulders, perpendicular to your body. Let your knees drop to your right side as you turn your head to the left. Try to keep both shoulders on the bed. Relax and hold for twenty seconds.

* Bring your knees and head back to center and repeat on the other side.

* Now that you're stretched and ready to start your day, it's time to get out of bed.

* Come on, get up!

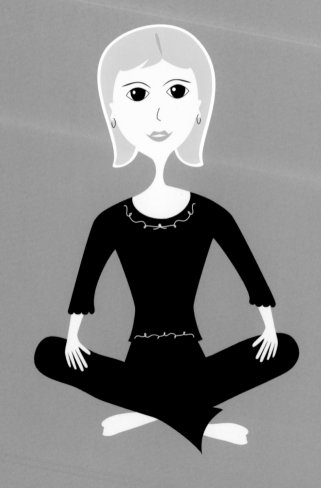

Glow-How

When the day gets hectic and you feel yourself slowly losing your composure, take a minute and remember your morning meditation. Bring your mind and body back to this quiet time. Allow yourself a moment to find your inner peace and balance; then return to your day calmer and more focused.

Set the tone of your day with a simple sunrise meditation. This special time devoted exclusively to you (just you, no kids or roommates or partners invited) will clear and calm your mind, focus your spirit, and relax your body. Spend just a few moments each morning in complete silence, and carry that calm, composed feeling with you for the rest of the day.

Silent Sunrise

* If you can manage it, get up before the rest of the household. This will allow you some quiet time that is really your own.

* Make sure your space is calm and peaceful. Remember, this meditation is meant to set the mood for the rest of the day.

* Sit cross-legged on the floor. Make sure you're comfortable; you may want a pillow for a little extra cushion. (If you have bad knees, it's probably best to grab a chair.) Sit up straight with your shoulders relaxed and down.

* Place your palms on your knees and slowly rock side to side, forward and backward, until you find your center and feel balanced.

* Rest your eyes comfortably on a spot in front of you. Keep your mouth relaxed and closed, and breathe evenly through your nose.

* Soak in the silence; listen to its quiet beauty; absorb its tranquillity. Your mind and body should be peaceful and steady, relaxed yet fully awake. Let any residual stress or tension dissipate as the silence cleanses your mind, body, and soul.

* Spend at least five minutes meditating, longer if you have the time.

* When you're done, thank yourself for this special time, slowly get up, and begin your day with focus and poise.

For more information on meditating, pick up a copy of *Glow Guide: Meditation.*

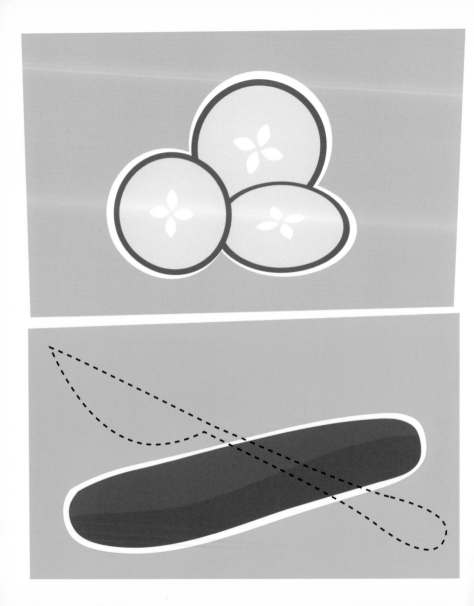

Cucumber is a wonderful cleanser and mild astringent that soothes the skin, fights wrinkles, and can even help bleach stubborn freckles. A quick cucumber mask is an easy morning treatment that will leave you feeling fresh-faced and ready to handle the day with a cool, composed ease.

Cool Cucumber Mask

* Start with a freshly washed face.

* Cut the cucumber into thin slices.

* Wet the washcloth with cool water and then wring it out.

* Lie down on the couch or your bed with your head and shoulders propped up just slightly, and place the cucumber slices on your face. Make sure you cover your entire face, including your eyes.

* Gently place the washcloth over the cucumber mask.

* Relax for about ten to fifteen minutes. Let your body drop away as your mind comes into sharp focus. Spend this time mentally preparing for the day. If you have a big presentation, imagine yourself walking in as cool as a cucumber. Big exam? No problem: see yourself skating right through it with icy precision. Breaking up with your boyfriend? Oh. Um, good luck.

* Slowly remove the washcloth and then dispose of the cucumbers.

* Splash your face with a bit of cool water and moisturize.

* Spend a moment admiring your fresh, radiant skin.

* Feel a sense of calm, cool collectedness about yourself. Carry this feeling for the rest of the day.

What You'll Need

1 cucumber

Knife

Washcloth

Cool water

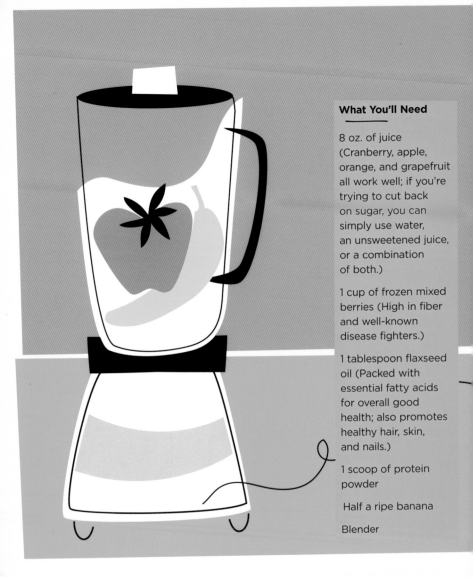

What You'll Need

8 oz. of juice (Cranberry, apple, orange, and grapefruit all work well; if you're trying to cut back on sugar, you can simply use water, an unsweetened juice, or a combination of both.)

1 cup of frozen mixed berries (High in fiber and well-known disease fighters.)

1 tablespoon flaxseed oil (Packed with essential fatty acids for overall good health; also promotes healthy hair, skin, and nails.)

1 scoop of protein powder

Half a ripe banana

Blender

A guilt-free pleasure that is also fast, easy, and nutritious, a fruit shake is a frosty treat. Skip the muffin this morning and try one for breakfast.

Sheer Smoothie Satisfaction

* Put all of the ingredients into a blender.

* Blend until smooth and creamy.

* Enjoy each sensational sip.

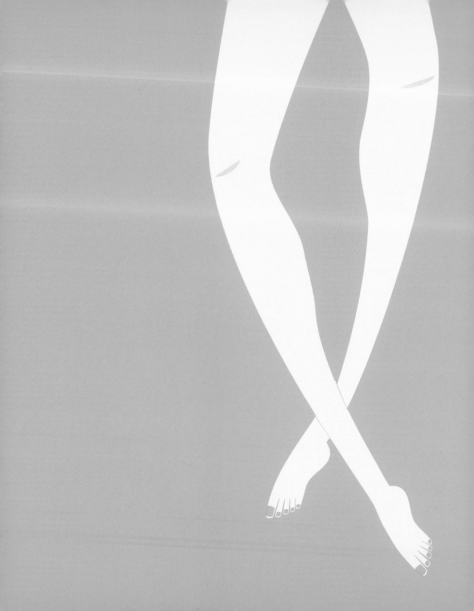

In the Nude

It's time to release your inner exhibitionist. Drop the towel and spend the morning in the buff. It's a liberating and invigorating way to bring in the day. Make your breakfast, read the paper, do some yoga, clean, whatever—just do it in the nude and give your body the chance to move freely and naturally. No restrictive waistbands or creeping undergarments, no sagging socks or uncomfortable shoes—you are as free and naked as a jaybird. Fly!

Glow-How

Give yourself some privacy and don't forget to close the blinds! Your neighbors may not be feeling quite as liberated as you.

Don't forget about your hands. They need love, too! Our hands and nails see a lot of action, yet very few of us give them the attention they need and deserve. Here's a quick and easy treatment you can squeeze in on your commute to work that will leave your hands and nails looking as good as they should.

Drive-Time Hand and Nail Treatment

* Massage the oil into your hands and nails. This stuff should glide on like butter.

* Carefully put on the gloves or socks and head off to work or school or wherever you're going.

* When you arrive, remove the gloves and rub in any excess oil.

If you're a little apprehensive about wearing socks on your hands in public, you can do this treatment at home, while watching TV, reading, sleeping, or talking on the phone. The idea is to keep the socks or gloves on for at least thirty minutes, or longer if possible, so fit it in whatever time slot your schedule allows.

What You'll Need

1 tablespoon sweet almond oil (rich in protein and emollients)

Cotton gloves or a pair of cotton socks

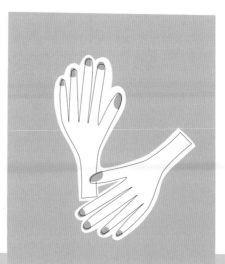

Glow-How

More treatments to show your hands a little love:

Brittle nails: After you wash your hands, rub a thick cream into your cuticles and nails. Try shea butter, which you can find at any health-food store. Be consistent; one time won't do it. Every time you wash, moisturize.

Yellow nails: Try a little lemon juice. Combine the juice of one lemon with a spoonful of olive oil. Soak your nails in this solution for ten to fifteen minutes twice a week until your nails are back to normal.

Rough skin: Wash your hands with a spoonful of sugar. (That's it—just sugar and water.) It will help gently scrub away dead skin and leave your hands soft and smooth.

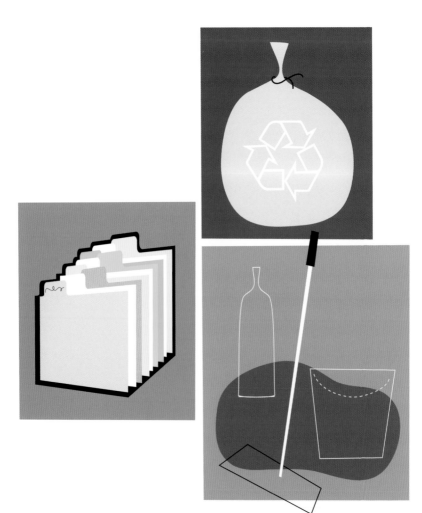

CHAPTER TWO

Daytime Detoxifiers

Our world is full of nasty stuff. Chemicals float around in the air, pesticides coat our food, clutter contaminates our space, toxic thoughts pollute our minds. In this chapter you will learn how to purge yourself, your environment, and your food of toxins and other unpleasant things. The exercises are simple and easy ways to clean your body, mind, and soul—top to bottom, inside and out. Cleanse your blood with a breathing exercise, stimulate your lymph system with a much-deserved massage, and clear your mind (and office) of clutter with an afternoon scrub and scour session. Whatever area of your life might need a good old-fashioned cleaning, this chapter's got just the supplies for you.

The state of your environment can drastically affect the state of your mind. If you're surrounded by chaos and disarray, chances are that's exactly how you feel. Taking a few moments to clear away clutter in your work space or living space will help clean up your mental space, too.

Cleaning for Clarity

* Throw out or recycle anything you don't need and put the rest away in its proper home.

* Organize bills, files, books, and magazines.

* Pull out the arsenal of cleaning supplies, some elbow grease, and get to work. Dust, wipe, sponge and sweep. Go crazy— cleaning can be very meditative and is a great way to release pent-up energy!

* When you're finished, sit down, take a deep breath, and enjoy the calm of a clean space and mind.

Green tea is well known for its powerful disease-fighting antioxidants, so drink it up! But don't throw out the tea bags—you can use those, too. When applied topically, green tea is an effective anti-inflammatory.

The Green Tea Two-in-One Treatment

* Brew two cups of green tea.

* Remove the tea bags from the tea and set them aside on a napkin. Give one cup of tea to your harried boss or roommate, and take one for yourself.

* Savor a sip of tea while you wait for the bags to cool off. (If you have access to a fridge, throw them in there for a few minutes.)

* When the bags have cooled, place them over your eyelids for ten minutes. This will help tighten your pores, calm your skin, and banish tired, puffy eyes.

* Sit back, relax, and breathe.

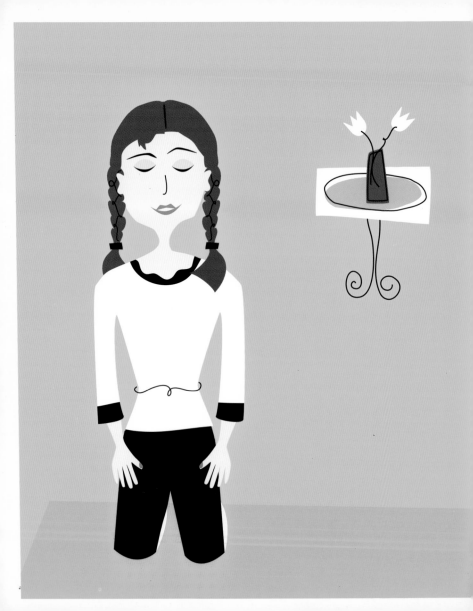

Negative thoughts (about yourself or others) are utterly unproductive and lead to nothing but stress, tension, and futility. Who needs that? Nobody. When these dubious opinions start to creep into your brain space (and from time to time, they will), here's a quick and easy way to kick them out.

Purge Toxic Thoughts

* Sit in your chair or cross-legged on the floor.

* Keep your back straight, your chin lifted, and your shoulders relaxed and down.

* Close your eyes.

* Place your palms on your knees or thighs.

* Take a deep breath in through your nose and, on the exhalation, release all of the negative thoughts occupying your brain. You feel fat today, you hate your job, your neighbor is annoying—let them all go.

* Now take a deep inhalation and breathe in the thoughts that make you feel good. You did well on a project, you're a great daughter, you're in love—whatever they may be, breathe them all in.

* Repeat this cycle until you've purged all of your toxic thoughts and your mind is filled with nothing but the positive.

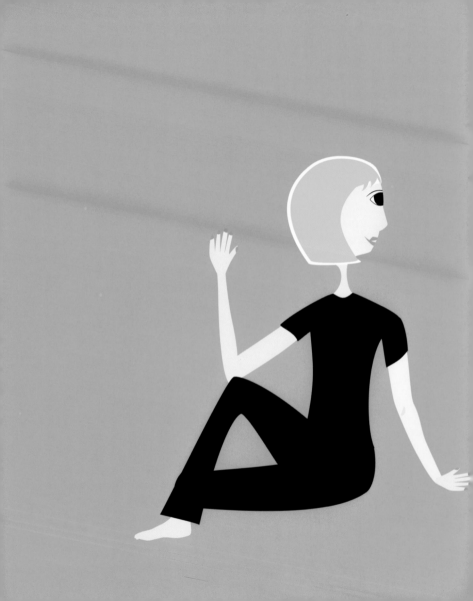

Spinal twists not only invigorate your mind and body, they also help remove toxins from your system. By aligning your spine and massaging your internal organs, a good spinal twist forces stubborn toxins out from their hiding places, allowing the body to whisk them away for elimination. With the amount of toxins you probably ingest on a daily basis (we all do; they're everywhere—car exhaust, secondhand smoke, food additives, cleaner fumes), do yourself a favor and stick in a spinal twist at least once a day.

Twist

* Sit on the floor with your legs extended straight out in front of you.

* Bend your right knee, bringing your right foot over your left leg so that it rests on the outside of your left knee. Now bend your left knee and pull your right foot toward you until it is next to your left thigh.

* Turn your torso to the right. Place your right hand on the ground next to you, arm straight. Bend your left arm at the elbow, bringing the elbow to the outside of your right knee.

* Keeping your back straight and your shoulders down, lift your chest, stretch your spine, and slowly, gently twist to the right. Use your left elbow as a leverage point, pushing it against your right knee. Turn your head to the right.

* Make sure your hips stay level and both sides of your buttocks remain on the ground.

* Really stretch. Feel your spine twisting. Groaning is fine and, is in fact, encouraged.

* Hold for three to five breaths, release, and switch sides.

Here are three simple but critical elements to ensure a detoxified system that you can easily make part of every day. They're free and readily available, so you have no excuses.

Detox Essentials

Water: There's lot of hype these days about drinking enough water. Here's a suggestion: believe the hype. Water is the *ultimate* detoxifier. It both cleans out and nourishes the body. Just eight glasses a day will help flush out built-up toxins, revive an overworked system, and sharpen a tired mind.

Exercise: When you exercise, you do two things: move and sweat. When you move, your lymph system is stimulated, helping your body carry waste away from your cells, and when you sweat, this waste is naturally released through your skin. Don't have time for a bona fide workout? A brisk walk around the block during lunch or in lieu of a coffee break will also do the trick.

Breath: Breathing supplies our bodies with oxygen, which both nourishes and cleanses our cells. The better we breathe, the more oxygen we take in, and the better we look and feel. Make a conscious effort to start breathing calmly, evenly, and deeply. You'll feel the difference in your mind, body, and soul. (See page 57 for a more detailed cleansing exercise.)

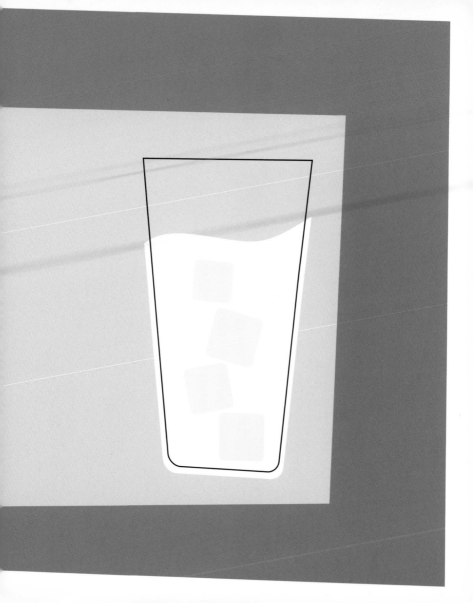

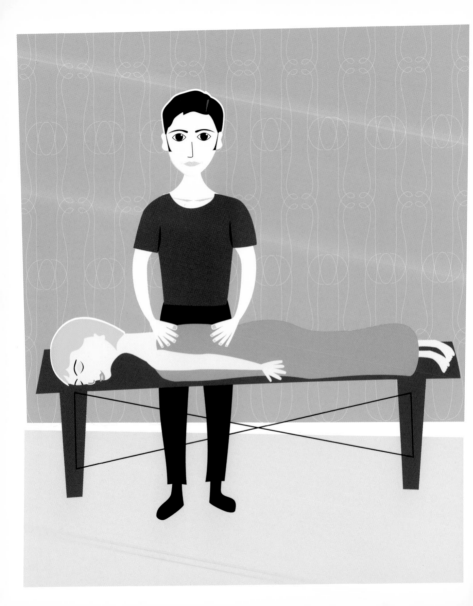

It's time to start prescribing yourself a monthly massage. Sure, it may seem like an indulgence, but really, it's more of a necessity. A good massage not only works out suppressed anxiety and tension, it also helps clean out the body. The lymph system is responsible for carrying metabolic waste away from your cells, and sometimes (because we're forced to sit around a lot) it gets backed up. During a massage, the lymph is loosened, allowing toxins to move more freely through and out of your body. So stop feeling guilty and schedule an appointment. It's good for your health. Really!

Rx: Massage

Swedish: A classic massage style. Your entire body is stroked, rubbed, and kneaded with light to medium pressure, helping to relax muscles, release tension, and stimulate blood flow and the lymphatic system.

Deep-Tissue: This type of massage takes a more aggressive approach, applying more intense pressure to release tension stored deep within the body.

Shiatsu: In this Japanese style (the name translates to "finger pressure") practitioners massage your energy meridians using their fingers, forearms, and elbows.

Reflexology: The foot has thousands of nerve endings, all of which, according to this Asian tradition, correspond with a part of the body. During a reflexology massage, points of the feet are stimulated to help release tension and encourage energy flow from other areas of the body.

Glow-How

Not sure what kind of massage to get? Check out this list of styles before you make your appointment.

Picture This

The next time stress and anxiety have gotten the best of you, instead of throwing a fit or dismembering your coworker, stop, close your eyes, take a deep breath, and visualize your favorite place—a scenic hiking trail, a pristine ski slope, a white sandy beach. See yourself there, feel the breeze on your face, the sand between your toes. Let the weight of the day fall away as you swish down the slopes or frolic in the surf.

Detox Lunch Box

Today, go organic. Give your body a break from preservatives, artificial coloring, pesticides, and chemicals, and eat a lunch of fresh, unadulterated food. You may find a smattering of organic fare at your local supermarket, but your best bet would be to swing by a health-food store or organic food market. There you will find a cornucopia of bright, beautiful fruits and veggies, and lots of other tasty stuff.

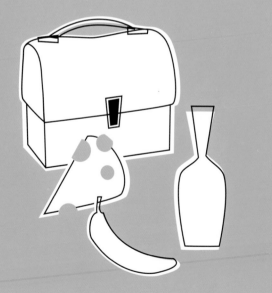

Glow-How

Unfortunately, organic food can get a little pricey. If you're on a budget, no big deal; you can still eliminate a good bit of the harmful stuff from your fruits and veggies with this simple soak. Combine 1/4 cup of hydrogen peroxide with two gallons of water. Bathe your produce in this solution for about twenty minutes, followed by a soak in a bath of plain water for an additional ten minutes. Dry off your goodies and enjoy.

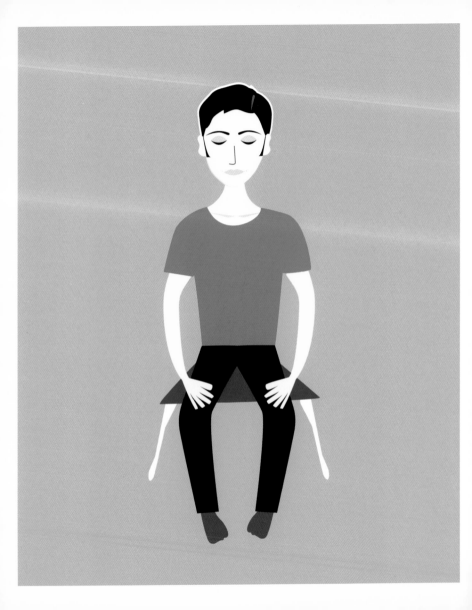

Bellows breath is a powerful breathing exercise that purifies the blood, improves the circulation, and enhances the energy flow throughout the body. When you're feeling overwhelmed and need to purge toxic stress and tension, forgo the break-down and instead opt for this cleansing technique.

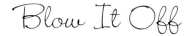

Blow It Off

* Sit in a chair with your back straight, your shoulders relaxed, and your feet planted on the ground. Place your palms on your knees.

* Do a deep exhalation through your nose. Feel your stomach muscles engage.

* Inhale and quickly exhale through your nose in sharp, repeated blasts. You don't need to consciously inhale again; your body will do that naturally. Just continue the rapid-fire exhalations.

* Feel your diaphragm's sharp movement as you blast, blast, blast air from your nose. Find a rhythm and don't hold your breath. Relax and let your natural breathing reflexes take over.

* Do ten rapid exhalations. Then take one deep breath in through your nose, hold it for a moment, and release it slowly and smoothly through your nose.

* Repeat the cycle.

CHAPTER THREE

Afternoon Revitalizers

Late day is usually when our energy and focus really start to wane, making it the perfect time to indulge in a quick spa treatment. This chapter provides the tools to help you treat yourself to some much-needed afternoon attention. Give your face a little lift with a facial massage. Stimulate your senses with a peppermint cold compress. Wake up a tired mind with a mist of cool rose water. This chapter is full of simple yet luxurious spa therapies to recharge your mind and body and revitalize your spirit.

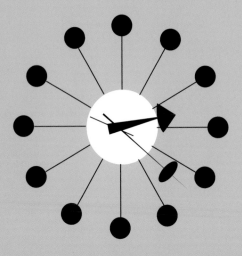

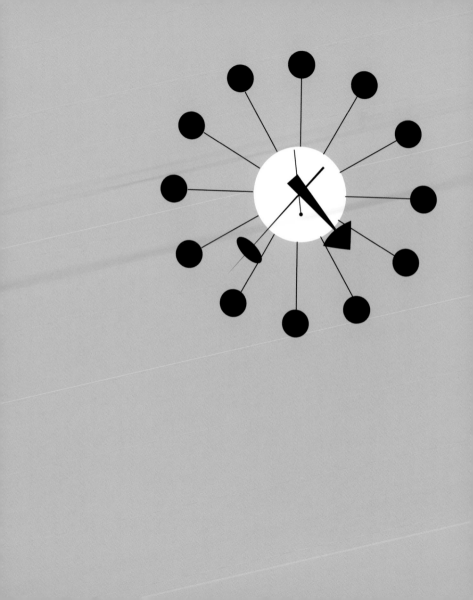

It is wise to keep a bowl of marbles on your desk or wherever you spend most of your time working or studying. While they can serve as a lovely aesthetic addition to your office or home decor, their more important function is to act as your personal reflexology masseuse. Put a handful under your desk and roll your feet over them. This will stimulate the reflex points on your soles, which will relax and invigorate your entire body.

Use Your Marbles

* Take off your shoes.

* Place a handful of marbles on the floor by your feet.

* Roll both feet slowly and firmly over the marbles.

* Your massage can go on for as long as you wish, but give yourself at least five minutes.

Glow-How

Using a golf ball will have the same effect. Make sure to stash one in your bag when you travel.

*Steal a moment between meetings or phone calls and give
yourself a quick facial massage. It's a simple way to ease tension.*

Face Lift

* Put a drop of geranium oil on the palms of your hands and rub
  it around. Cup each hand slightly, and gently place your palms
  over your face, on either side of your nose.

* Close your eyes and breathe deeply. Relax. The scent should
  help relieve and calm a chaotic mind.

* Now bring your first two fingers to the inside of your eyebrow
  line and make a sideways peace sign, placing your index finger
  just under your eyebrow and your middle just under your eye.
  Moving from the inside out, sweep the eye socket, stopping at
  the temple. Don't push too hard; you don't want to stretch the
  skin. Apply firm but gentle pressure.

* Repeat this a few times and then stop again at the temple.
  With your index and middle fingers together and on your
  temples, begin to move your fingers in a forward circular motion.
  The skin should move with your fingers. Do ten rotations.

* Leaving your first two fingers on your temples, bring your
  thumbs to the inside of your cheekbones. Applying pressure
  underneath the bone with the thumbs, gently work your way
  back out to your temples. Repeat.

* Bring your fingers to your chin. Pinch the chin with the thumb
  and fingers. Hold for a moment, and then repeat, moving out
  along the jawline. When you reach the end of your jaw, work your
  way back to your chin. Hold for a moment and release.

* Put four fingers of one hand together and place them on your forehead, parallel to your brow. Sweep your fingers up from the brow line into your hairline. Move from the right to the left temple. When you reach the left temple, sweep back toward the right.

* Bring your fingertips to your scalp. Working from your hairline to your neck, massage your scalp in circular motions.

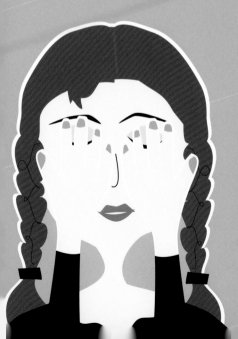

Refreshing your mind and body after a marathon morning of meetings and deadlines is easy: wash your face. Don't have a mild facial soap handy? No problem—just grab some honey. This amazing cleanser has been used as a skin treatment since Cleopatra's day.

Egyptian Cleanser

* Wet your face and massage the honey into your skin.

* Move your fingers in circular motions from your chin up to your forehead.

* Rinse well.

* Close pores with a splash of cold water.

* Moisturize.

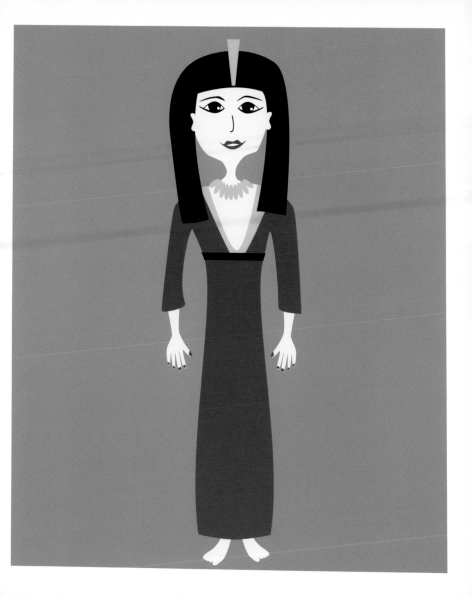

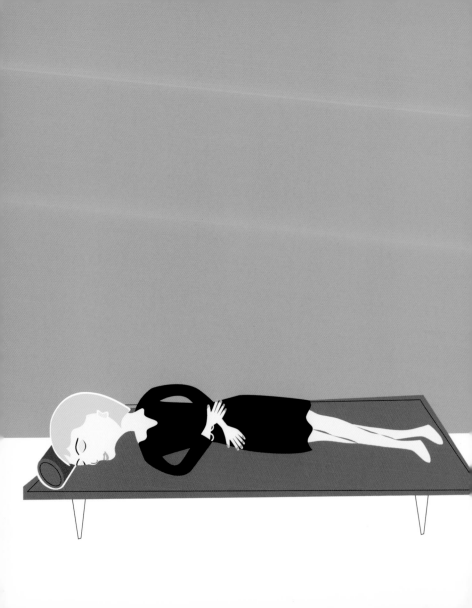

If you're worn out, allow yourself a few stolen moments to nap. Stress shoots your blood pressure up, forcing your heart to work harder. And when your heart has to work harder, it wears the rest of you out. Taking a nap helps you slow down, allowing your blood pressure to drop and your body a chance to revitalize.

Snooze

* Find a quiet spot. (Your bed is ideal, but a couch, a park bench, or that dark spot under your desk will do.)

* Get prone and relax.

* Try to rest for at least fifteen minutes, but shoot for thirty.

* Don't feel the slightest bit guilty. Enjoy every restful second— you deserve it.

Grumpy? Irritated? Throwing out nasty glances and curt remarks? What a waste of energy! Instead of squandering your vibes on negativity, start sending out some of the positive variety. Not only does it show respect for yourself and others, but practicing loving-kindness will also lift your spirits and boost your energy.

Be Kind

* Bring your frazzled boss a cup of tea.

* Write your grandfather a letter.

* Remind your best friend of her most stellar quality.

* Talk to a stranger.

* Give the grumpy bus driver a well-deserved pat on the back.

* And don't forget to treat yourself! Buy a big bouquet of wildflowers for your desk or schedule yourself an early-evening pedicure.

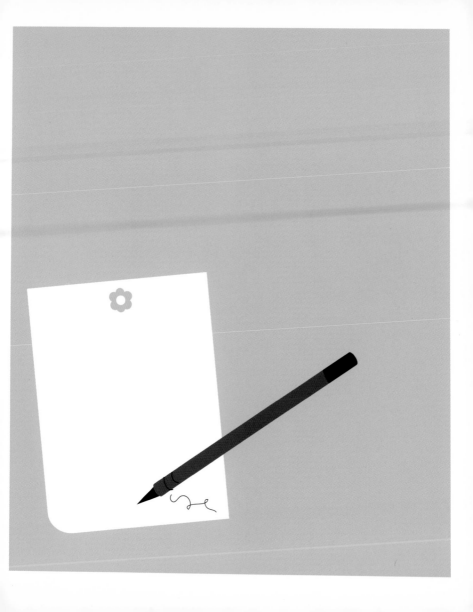

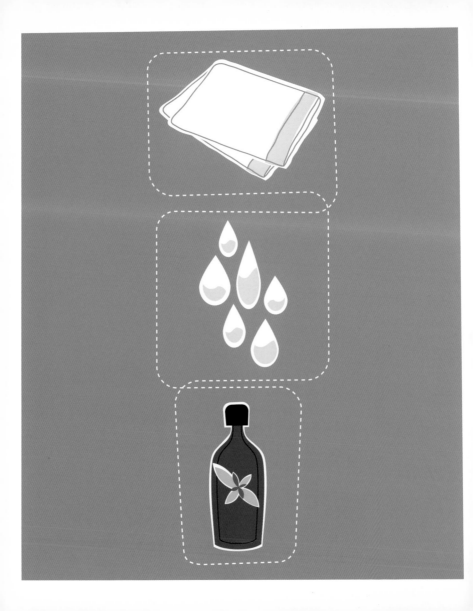

Placing a cold compress on the back of your neck is a quick and easy way to invigorate the body and soul. It increases blood flow to your brain, upping your energy while leaving you feeling refreshed and renewed. For an even greater stimulant, dilute some peppermint oil and sprinkle a few drops on your compress.

Peppermint Compress

* Grab a washcloth and soak it in cold water.

* Ring it out and fold it into a rectangle.

* Sprinkle a few drops of diluted peppermint oil on the compress.

* Sit down. Relax and let your head and neck hang forward.

* Place the cold compress on the back of your neck.

* Relax and enjoy for ten minutes.

Staring at a computer screen or textbook all day can wreak havoc on your eyes. Here's a quick exercise to relieve eyestrain and strengthen your eye muscles.

Tired-Eye Treatment

* Sit in a chair or cross-legged on the floor. Make sure your back and neck are straight and your shoulders are relaxed and down. Place your left palm on your left knee. Get comfortable.

* Straighten the index and middle finger of your right hand, gently folding the remaining fingers into your palm.

* Extend your right arm out in front of you, your palm facing up. Relax your face.

* Focus your eyes and mind on your extended fingers; let everything else fade away.

* Slowly and steadily move your fingers toward your face, following them with your eyes. Gently touch your nose, letting your eyes roll inward. Hold for a moment.

* Return your arm to its starting position, again maintaining your focus.

* Keeping your face forward and your head and neck still but not rigid, move your fingers up and to the right, and slowly down in a diagonal line to your lower left. Continue following with your eyes.

* Now move your fingers up and left, then slowly in a diagonal to your lower right.

* Repeat with your left hand.

* Now close your eyes for a moment. Let them relax and soak in the benefits of the exercise.

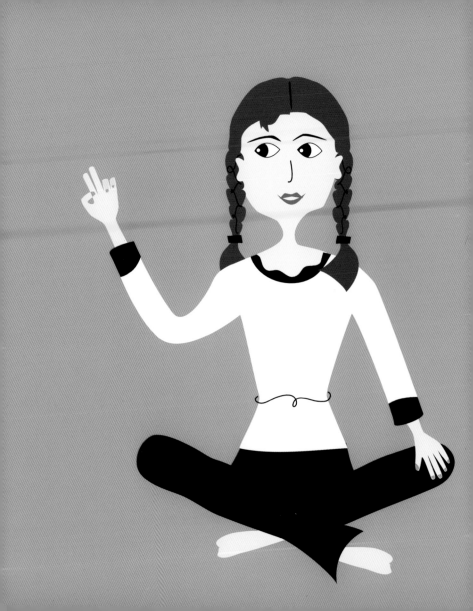

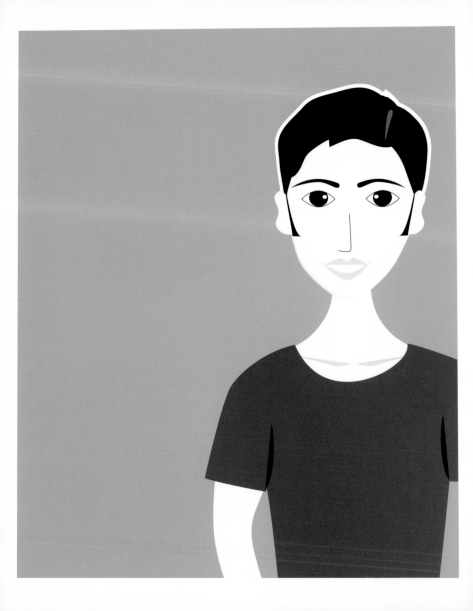

Smiling, even when you don't feel like it, can radically revitalize your mood. It brings a lift to your face and a boost to your soul. Not convinced? Try it. You'll be pleasantly surprised.

Smile!

* Close your eyes and relax your face. Breathe deeply.

* Slowly start to smile. If you feel an inner resistance to smiling, do it anyway!

* Now send your smile to the rest of your body—down your neck; into your chest, back, and arms; down your legs. Feel your body start to radiate as your smile emanates from every pore.

* Smiling is contagious. Smile at friends, coworkers, strangers, and see how quickly it catches on.

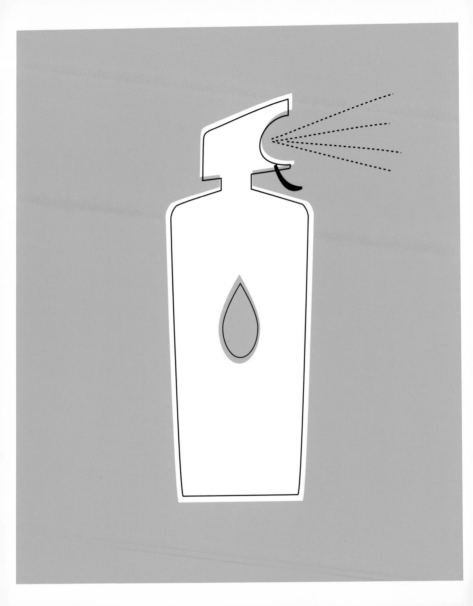

Feeling a little run down? Stop and smell the roses. A simple blast of rose water, a mild antiseptic toner, will soothe and refresh your skin and liven up your soul. Chill it beforehand for an even more invigorating effect.

Rose-Water Rejuvenator

* Fill a clean spray bottle with rose water and store it in the refrigerator. (You can find rose water at most grocery or health-food stores.)

* When you need a quick pick-me-up, grab the bottle, settle into your chair, close your eyes, and mist your face.

* Take a deep breath and spend the next few moments relaxing and recharging.

* Open your eyes refreshed and renewed.

Glow-How

If you're still feeling wiped out, it's time for a little acupressure. Pinch the fleshy area between your thumb and index finger for one to two minutes. This is said to give your body a quick dose of energy.

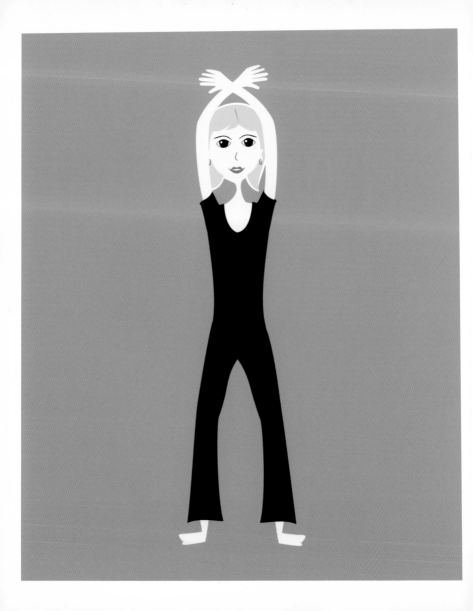

T'ai Chi is an ancient Chinese movement meditation. Its slow, deliberate movements calm the breathing, clear the mind, and relax the body. The idea behind this centuries-old practice is to release tension and blocked energy so that your body can move freely from your dan tien, or center of gravity. When your body is in sync with gravity, your movements become effortless, and as a result, you have more energy. If you want to learn more about T'ai Chi, your best bet would be to take a class—this art form can get a bit complicated. But first get acquainted with the practice through the simple exercise below. The trick: let each movement flow into the next.

Slow Motion

* Stand with your feet slightly apart, your weight evenly distributed on both soles, your knees soft.

* Take a deep breath and on the exhalation, feel all stress and tension leave your body. Let everything go.

* Bring your arms up in front of your body, parallel to the floor. They should be straight but not locked or rigid.

* Slowly exhale, lowering your arms and crossing them in front of you, right hand under left, simultaneously bending your knees.

* Inhale, and in a sweeping motion, raise your crossed arms up in front of your face and over your head as you straighten your knees.

* Slowly separate your arms, creating an arch over your head; then turn your palms outward.

* Exhale as you continue to lower your outstretched arms. Bend your knees as you bring your arms down and back around, crossing them in front of you.

* Finish as you began, with your right hand underneath your left and your knees bent.

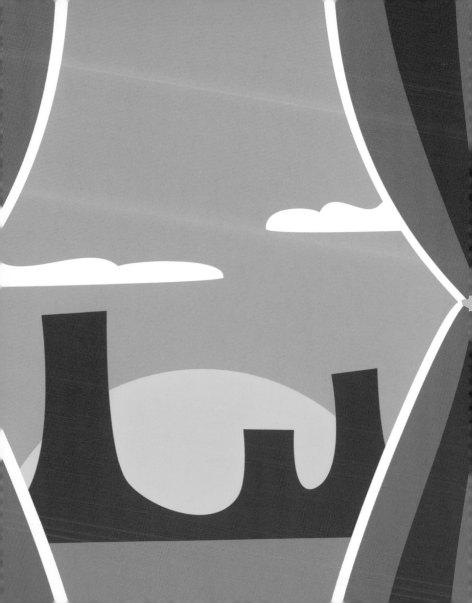

CHAPTER FOUR

Evening Relaxers

After an arduous day, it can be hard to unwind. But learning how to release stress is an important part of maintaining health and happiness. The treatments and exercises in this chapter will school you in relaxation techniques that help loosen stubborn tension so you can really let it go. Whether it's a hot rock massage, a little music therapy, or a sunset stroll, this chapter's got whatever you need to settle into a relaxing evening. So tonight, turn off the television, push the bills aside, put the laundry back in the hamper, and use the time instead to take care of you, and only you.

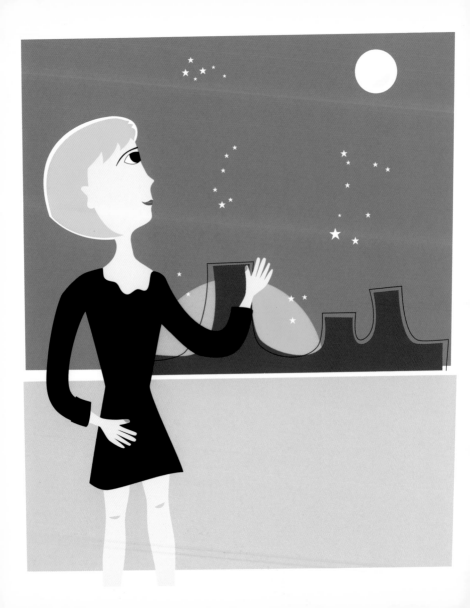

Dusk is the perfect time for a mindful walk. Just as the sun is winding down its day (at least in our hemisphere), so are you. Take this time to walk off any lingering stress or anxiety, and bask in the warm glow of the setting sun.

Sunset Stroll

* Put down your Walkman; this is quiet time. No music or talk radio. It's just you, your breath, and the great outdoors.

* Slow down and take it easy. This walk is meant to calm you down, not rev you up. Don't think about where you're going or how far you've gone—simply walk.

* Breathe slowly, deeply, and rhythmically.

* Take notice of your body and how it feels; home in on any tense spots and try to release them.

* Forget about the pile of work on your desk or the fight you had with your boss. With each step, let it all go.

* Pay attention to the surroundings. Notice the trees and sky; stop for a moment and smell a rose or touch its petals. Listen to the birds or the wind.

* Continue walking mindfully for thirty minutes.

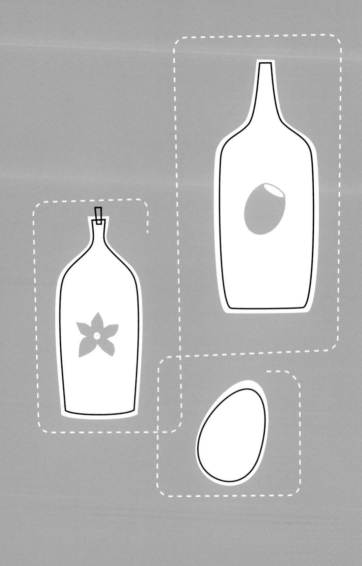

There's no need to go to an expensive spa for a facial when you can just as easily take matters into your own hands at home. And more than skin therapy, an evening facial will give you some solo time to relax and reengage with yourself.

Full-Service Facial

* Clean. Remove your makeup. (Out of makeup remover? Grab some olive oil. It's a great natural alternative.) Wash your face with a gentle cleanser. (Whole milk and yogurt are wonderful soap substitutes.)

* Steam. Give yourself a steam. (See page 21 for instructions.) Add a few drops of essential oil to the water for added benefits. Choose eucalyptus to fight oil, jasmine to calm irritated skin, and geranium to moisturize.

* Exfoliate. Using your preferred exfoliating scrub (or simply add a spoonful of sugar, cornmeal, poppy seeds, or finely ground almonds to a spoonful of honey), start at your neck and in circular motions work your way up to your forehead. Take your time and be present with yourself and aware of your movements.

* Rinse thoroughly.

* Mask. Cover your face with a thick layer of mashed avocado for dry skin, scrambled raw egg for oily skin, or mayonnaise for normal skin. Sit back and relax for about twenty minutes. Rinse well.

* Throw on some light moisturizer and you're done.

Glow-How

If you must pop your pimples, do so after you exfoliate, before applying the mask. And for goodness' sake, be gentle and don't use your nails! Wiggle the little sucker out of there; don't pry it. If it won't budge, leave it alone. You'll only make matters bigger—and redder.

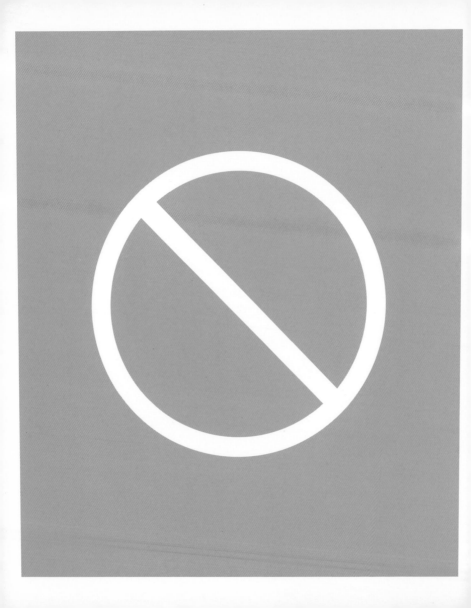

Give your mind and body a break from moving and thinking and reacting. Don't lift a finger, don't watch TV, don't talk, and don't even think about loading the dishwasher or mopping the floor. This is a special time when you will do absolutely nothing.

Doing nothing is actually a lot harder than it sounds. Here are a few suggestions to help you come to a complete stop.

Do Nothing

* Find a secluded area away from your roommates or family where you can sit in silence and relax.

* Turn off the television and radio, and unplug the phone.

* Make sure the mail and today's paper are both out of sight.

* Plop down and let yourself sink into a chair or the floor or wherever you choose to sit. Don't think, don't move; just sit. Resist the urge to get up, and don't feel guilty for "wasting time." This is a productive time spent nurturing your mind, body, and soul. Revel in it.

After a long day, relieve sore feet and relax a frazzled mind with an herb-infused foot soak. And for kicks, top it off with a pedicure. Your feet will look and feel like new.

Herbal Foot Soak

* Heat up the water in the pot. Add the marjoram (which is known to relax and calm the mind and body), Epsom salts, and baking soda, and allow to simmer for a few minutes.

* While you're waiting, remove any nail polish from your toes, wash your feet, and gather together all of the tools you'll need for your pedicure.

* Pour the water into the basin, sit down, ease your feet in, and relax for ten minutes. Read a magazine or a book of poetry, listen to music, or just sit in silence.

* While your feet are still in the water, use the pumice stone to rub away any dead skin or calluses on your toes and heels. (See page 119 for a special callus cure.)

* Remove your feet from the water and pat them dry.

* Using an orange stick, gently push your cuticles back, but don't cut them.

* Trim or file your nails to a desired length.

* Massage your feet with a thick cream. Don't skimp on the massage. Reflexology is a great stress and tension reliever.

* Wipe any excess cream from your nails.

* This time skip the polish and go au naturel. Dab your nails with a bit of mineral oil and buff them until they shine.

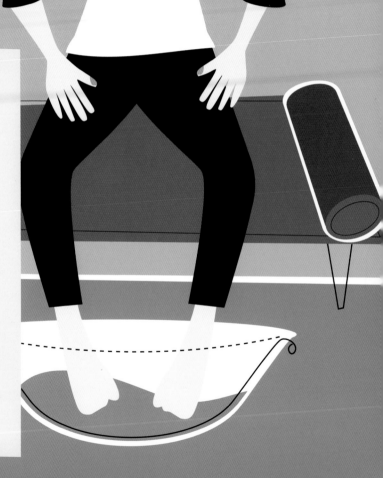

What You'll Need

2 gallons of water

Pot

2 cups dried marjoram

½ cup Epsom salts

½ cup baking soda

Foot basin

Pumice stone

Towel

Orange stick

Nail file or clipper

Thick cream

Mineral oil

Nail buffer

Invade your rock garden and indulge in this deeply therapeutic body massage adapted from the centuries-old Native American tradition.

Hot Rock Massage

* Place the rocks in the pot and fill it with water until they are totally submerged. Let the water come to a full boil, then turn off the heat. After the water has cooled for ten to fifteen minutes, drain it. The rocks should be warm but not too hot.

* Dry the rocks with the towel and find a cozy place to sit. Make sure you have enough room to extend your legs and you don't feel cramped.

* Cover the smaller stones with tea tree oil and place one between each toe. Tea tree oil is well known for its ability to fight bacteria and will help keep your feet free of—gasp!—athlete's foot.

* Place a few drops of jojoba oil on one of the larger rocks and rub it around. Starting at your ankles, rub the rock up and down your legs in long, smooth strokes. Don't push too hard. Be gentle with yourself.

* Move to your abdomen and chest, again using long, smooth, gentle strokes. Then continue on to your shoulders, neck, and finally each arm.

* Feel the heat from the stone ease tense muscles and sooth away any pent-up stress and anxiety.

* Pick up the other large rock so you are holding one in each hand. Lie down on your back with your arms slightly out from your sides and your palms up. Starting at your feet and moving up to your head, slowly relax every one of your muscles. Give yourself at least ten minutes to enjoy this total relaxation.

* When you're ready, set the larger stones aside and remove the small stones from your toes. Rub the excess tea tree oil into your feet.

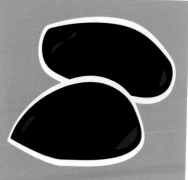

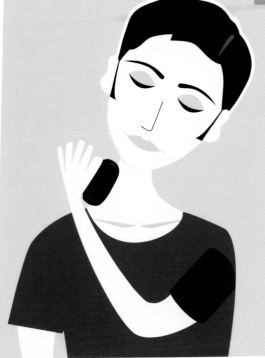

What You'll Need

———

2 large, smooth, flat rocks

8 small stones (but large enough to fit snugly between your toes)

Pot

Water

Towel

Tea tree oil

Jojoba oil

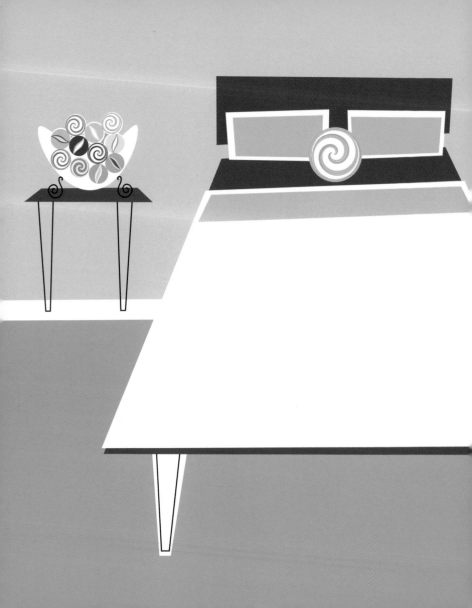

Feng shui is the study of energy flow—more specifically, how the flow of energy (what the Chinese call chi) *in your environment affects the flow of your personal* chi. *The art of feng shui is learning to sync up these energies to create a more harmonious home and a more harmonious you. Your bedroom is where your* chi *is rested and rejuvenated, so there are a few special pains you should take to orient the room for optimum relaxation. Here's how:*

Bedroom Feng Shui

* The ideal purpose of your bedroom is to sleep, so make your bed the focus of the room. If you're sleeping on an old or used mattress, it may be time to indulge in a new one. The condition of your bed is very important to cultivating positive *chi*. A new bed will bring with it new energy.

* Try to use the room for its primary purpose: rest and relaxation. Haul out the TV, stereo, and any other electronic devices. Oh, and the phone goes, too. This is meant to be a quiet, peaceful place for your mind and body.

* Get rid of any clutter; it blocks energy flow. Remove stacks of books or magazines, piles of clothes, and any unnecessary furniture. Think sparse and simple.

* Clean, clean, clean. A clean room ushers in fresh, clean energy.

* Now your bedroom is oriented for optimum rest. Sweet dreams.

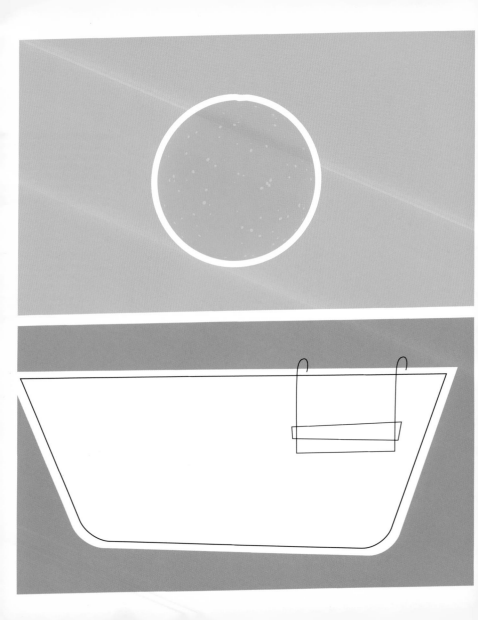

A renowned feng shui cure for reviving and restoring personal chi, *an evening orange-peel bath is a great way to relax and unwind. Give it a try when you feel your positive vibes starting to wane.*

Orange-Peel Cure

* Draw a bath.

* Place the peels of nine oranges in the water. (According to tradition, the number nine symbolizes power and will make the cure more potent, and the oranges themselves are known for their reviving and purifying properties.) Don't let the remaining oranges go to waste. Eat one and use the rest to make some freshly squeezed juice.

* Slide in, sit back, and relax. Feel your energy being restored as you soak in the revitalizing properties of the orange peel.

* When you've had a good soak, get out of the bath, dry off, and slip into your robe. It's time to top off the cure with the Three Secrets of Reinforcement, a technique said to help strengthen the cure.

* Simply put your hands in prayer position (the body secret), repeat your favorite mantra nine times (the speech secret), and visualize yourself with renewed energy, vibrant and full of life (the mind secret). This all might seem a little odd, but you've got nothing to lose, so why not give it a try. You may even find that this little ritual brings you not only renewed energy but also a sense of calm and a feeling of well-being.

After a difficult day, a simple nighttime meditation will give you a chance to slow down, clear your head, and release any lingering tension and stress. Not only will it calm your mind and relax your body, but it will also give you a few precious moments of much-needed silence and solitude.

Evening Meditation

* Light a stick of incense and place it a few feet in front of you.

* Sit on the floor with your legs crossed (you may want a pillow for a little extra cushioning) and shift your body around until you are centered and comfortable.

* Keeping your spine straight and your shoulders relaxed, place your palms on your knees.

* Rest your eyes on the burning incense or simply on a spot in front of you. Close your mouth and breathe through your nose. Breathe deeply and evenly.

* Focus on the scent of the incense and let all outside distractions fall away. The pile of work on your desk, the fight with your partner, the hamper full of laundry in your bedroom—let it all go. This time is for you and you only.

* When you're ready, thank yourself for this quiet time and slowly get up.

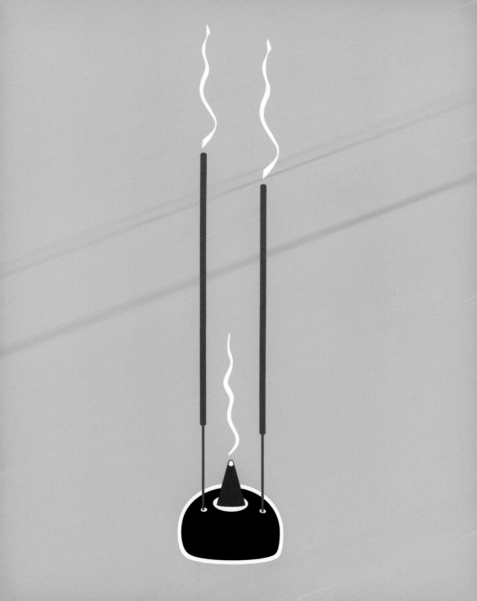

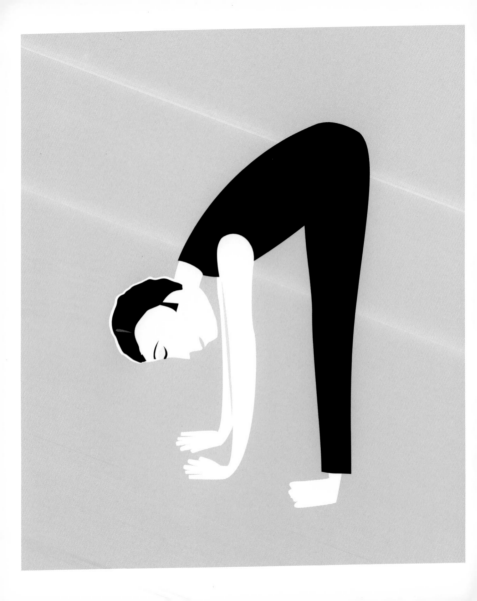

Folding into a simple forward bend will slow your heart rate, calm your mind, and ease tension stored in your lower back and hamstrings. Spend just a few moments in this relaxation posture and feel the weight of the day slip from your fingertips.

Bend a little

* Stand with your feet together. Breathe in deeply and lift your arms over your head.

* Slowly exhale and fold your body forward. Let your torso and arms relax and hang loose. If you can touch the ground, place your palms on the floor in front of you. If you're not terribly flexible and can't quite reach the floor, just let your arms dangle or rest them on your calves or ankles.

* Breathe slowly, deeply, and evenly for five breaths. (One inhalation and one exhalation equals one breath.)

* Slowly roll your body up one vertebra at a time, lifting your head up last.

Chill tunes soothe the soul and massage a tired mind. Tonight, take a few moments to kick back and listen to your favorite moody music. Feel stress and anxiety fade into the background as your body relaxes to the rhythms and beats.

Music Therapy

* Throw in a CD, something soothing and melodious.

* Absorb the sound.

* Feel the rhythm roll through your body, relaxing every muscle, joint, and organ.

* Tap your foot, swing your hips; let the positive energy of the music course through your mind, body, and soul.

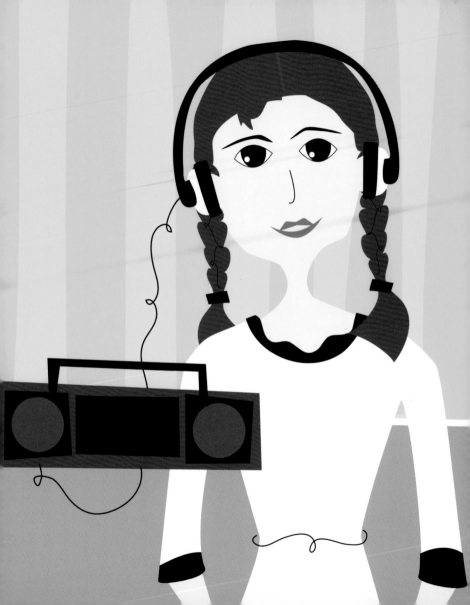

While the rest of the world is asleep, wash away lingering stress and anxiety, unnecessary emotions, and negative energy, and soak in the silence and solitude. Add a little neroli oil, a natural sedative derived from the bitter orange tree, to really unwind.

Midnight Bath

* Dim the lights and light a candle.

* Following the Japanese tradition, give yourself a quick rinse in the shower to remove the day's grime before your bath.

* Draw the bath. Keep the temperature somewhere around 100 degrees. Add the oatmeal and baking soda, two skin-soothing ingredients, and the neroli oil.

* Slip into the tub. Spend some time just soaking. Feel tense muscles start to relax. Enjoy the utter silence.

* Imagine the water gently flowing through your body, cleansing it of stress and anxiety. Feel the water running down your neck, shoulders, and arms, into your chest, back, and abdomen, rushing into your legs and feet, and finally pouring out your fingers and toes.

* Let any tension and negative emotions dissolve into the water.

What You'll Need

Candle

2 cups oatmeal

1 cup baking soda

6 drops neroli oil

Glow-How

If you prefer to use dried herbs rather than oil, put them in a tea ball or a muslin drawstring bag. You'll need one to two cups. Here is a list of herbs you may want to try:

Bergamot: helps ease depression and refresh the mind and body

Chamomile: well known for its sedative properties

Clary sage: relaxes the muscles

Peppermint: stimulates the body and soul

Rosemary: boosts energy and helps decongest

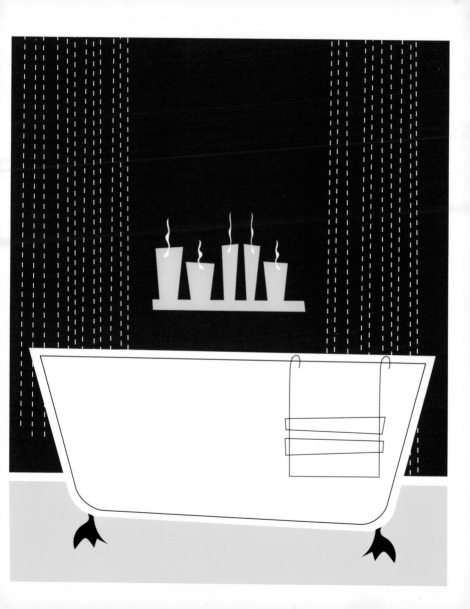

CHAPTER FIVE

Overnight Rejuvenators

Sleeping is an intrinsic time of renewal, when the mind and body are naturally restored and refreshed, but that doesn't mean you can't help things along. You can, and this chapter will show you how. It is packed with treatments that work while you sleep. Whether you need to remove product buildup from your hair, get rid of stubborn calluses, condition dry cracked lips, or banish blemishes, this clever chapter shows you how to use those resting hours for more than just a good snooze.

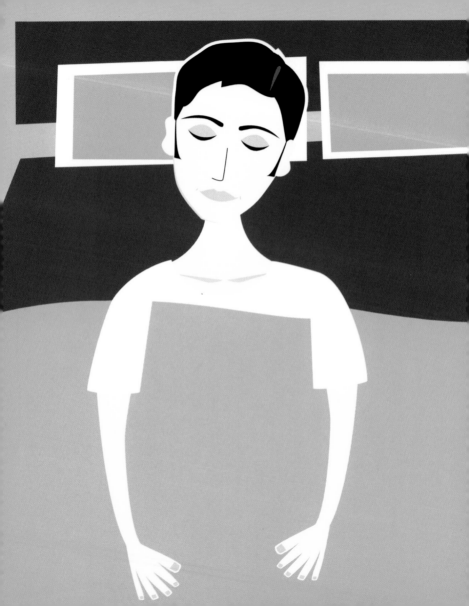

Sleep is the number one overnight rejuvenator—eight hours devoted solely to rest and renewal. More than any cream, toner, or treatment, a solid sleep does wonders not only for your complexion but for the health and well-being of your mind, body, and soul. Here are a few tips for getting a good night's rest.

Sleep!

* Exercise, exercise, exercise. An afternoon jog in the park or an early evening walk will help you release any pent-up energy, stress, or anxiety, so you can sleep more soundly. (Make sure you work out sometime during the day. Waiting until late at night can make it difficult to fall asleep.)

* Avoid caffeine and alcohol in the evening. Even the slightest amount can disrupt an otherwise restful sleep.

* Take a warm bath. You'll be more than ready for bed after a thirty-minute soak.

* Meditate. A little late-night meditation will help you slow down, clear your mind of the day's tedium, and thoroughly relax your body.

* Have a cup of chamomile tea. It has long been known for its relaxing and tranquilizing effects.

Glow-How

Use the weekend to catch up on sleep you may have lost through-out the week. And don't feel guilty—sleeping in is good for you!

Ditch those ratty sheets and that lone, lumpy pillow; you deserve an upgrade. Transform an ordinary bed into an oasis of rest and rejuvenation with a few simple but sumptuous additions.

Feather Your Nest

Suggested adornments for your new sleeping sanctuary:

* New 100 percent cotton sheets (or, at the minimum, freshly washed sheets)

* Lots and lots of pillows

* A chenille or cashmere blanket, or something equally soft and snuggly

* A cotton or down duvet

* An egg-crate foam pad or feather bed

* More pillows!

* New PJs

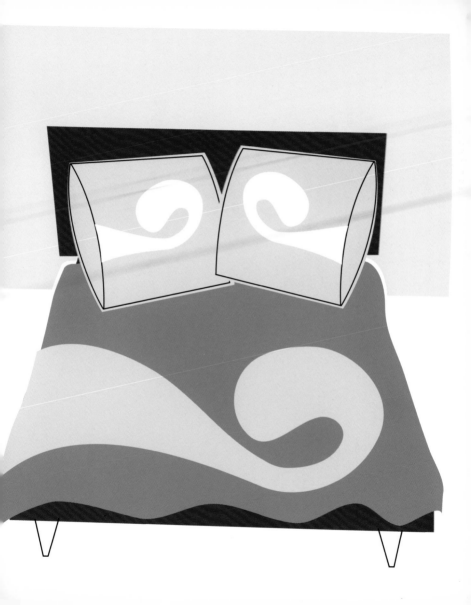

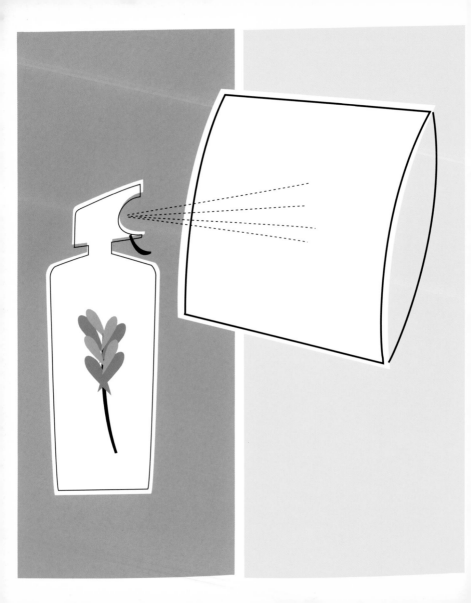

Before you hit the sheets, mist your pillow with the delicate scent of lavender. This natural sedative will help you relax and drift off into a deep and restful sleep.

Lavender Pillow Mist

* Pour the water, witch hazel, and lavender oil into the spray bottle.

* Replace the bottle's top, making sure it is tightened securely, and shake vigorously.

* Mist your pillow.

* Crawl into bed and breathe in the soothing scent of lavender. Feel your mind, body, and soul fall away as you fade into a deep sleep.

What You'll Need

½ cup water

½ teaspoon witch hazel

4 to 5 drops lavender essential oil

Small spray bottle

Glow-How

Make sure to pack your lavender mist when you travel! It will help turn an otherwise stale hotel into a sweet-smelling haven of peaceful sleep.

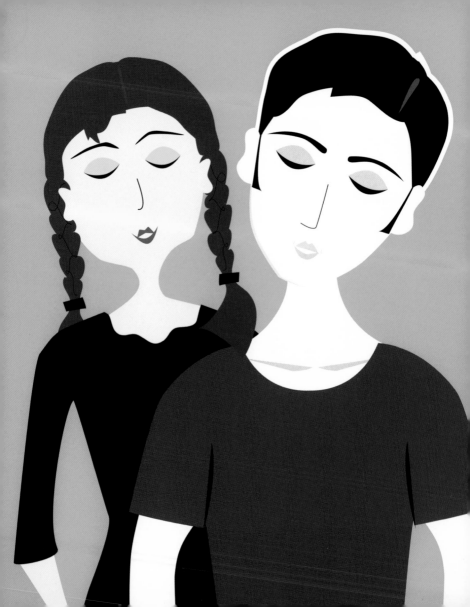

Lip Service

The lips see a lot of action during the day and night—eating, drinking, talking, laughing, and if you're lucky, kissing—and just like any other part of an overworked body, they deserve some attention, too. Before bed, pamper your pout with a little coconut oil (a solid white oil found at the grocery store that is great at holding in moisture). Apply a layer after you brush your teeth, and wake up in the morning with soft, smooth, conditioned lips.

Glow-How

If you have dry, flaky lips, gently rub them with a soft-bristle toothbrush to exfoliate the dead skin before you apply the oil.

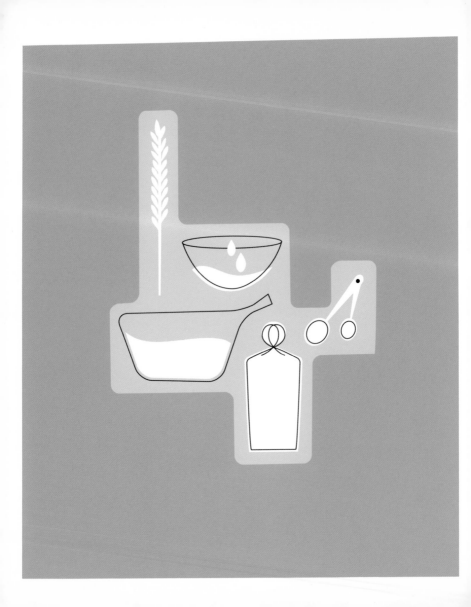

After an evening bath or shower, take an extra minute before you crawl into bed and rub yourself down with this rich, heavy cream. It will lock in moisture and rehydrate your skin as you sleep. (This is also a good time to give yourself a little massage.)

Overnight Body Butter

What You'll Need

---

1 tablespoon coconut oil

1/4 cup grated cocoa butter

3 tablespoons wheat germ oil

1 tablespoon grated beeswax

Small glass bowl

Pan

Water

Small glass container

* Put all of the ingredients in a small, shallow glass bowl.

* Fill the pan with two inches of water and warm with low heat.

* Place the bowl in the pan. When the wax melts, gently stir the ingredients together.

* Pour the cream into the small glass container and let cool.

* When the mixture has cooled completely, gently stir it again.

* Apply the cream to your body after your evening shower or bath.

* Awake to soft, supple skin.

Gel, mousse, hair spray—the product list could go on and on—get massaged into our hair every day. They lift, they hold, they style, but they also leave a thin layer of residue. Eventually that residue turns into a bone fide buildup, and our once bouncy, shiny tresses become dull and lifeless. Here's a quick and easy hair treatment that will remove the buildup and return your locks to their natural sheen.

Buildup Buster

* Wet your hair.

* Gently towel-dry, then comb out any tangles.

* Massage the peanut oil into your hair, distributing it evenly from the roots to the ends.

* Put on the shower cap or hair turban and hit the sack.

* In the morning, shampoo your hair as you normally would and style as usual. Notice the return of your hair's natural body and shine.

What You'll Need

Towel

2 tablespoons peanut oil

Shower cap or hair turban

Had a bit of a breakout today? No problem. Let a little vitamin A–packed egg yolk take care of those pesky pimples while you sleep.

Zit Zapper

* Wash your face and pat dry.

* Moisturize as you normally would, but avoid the problem area.

* Dab a bit of yolk on the blemish; let it dry, and dream that pimple away.

Glow-How

A dab of tea tree oil, a natural antiseptic, also helps relieve blemishes. And if you have any residual scarring or discoloration from past breakouts, a spot of wheat germ oil (high in vitamins A and E) will help the healing process along.

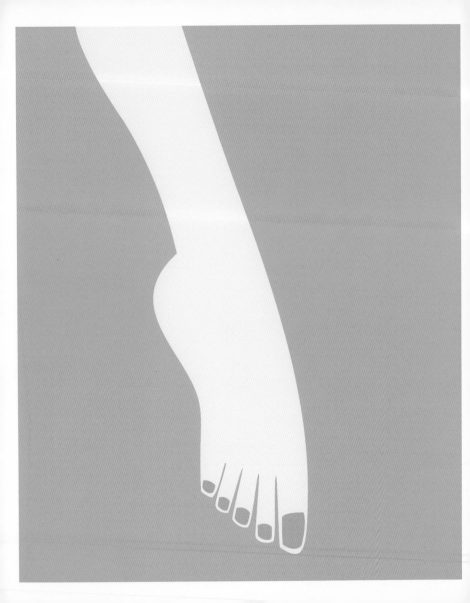

Feet looking a little bit weathered? Don't fret. You can banish unsightly calluses and rough skin with this easy overnight treatment. It will leave your feet and toes soft, smooth, and beautiful. So throw those combat boots aside—it's time for some strappy sandals.

Callus Cure

What You'll Need

Towel

Liquid wart remover (Sounds gross, but believe me, you'll love the results.)

Heavy moisturizer or Vaseline

Cotton socks

Pumice stone

* Wash your feet and pat them dry.

* Apply the wart remover to any calluses or rough patches and allow to dry.

* Cover your feet with a heavy moisturizer (Vaseline also works well) and carefully put on the socks.

* Sleep while this treatment works its magic.

* In the morning, take a shower and *gently* rub off the calluses and rough skin with the pumice stone. See how easily they slough off and how smooth and soft your feet have become.

* Dry your feet and moisturize.

* Treat yourself to a new pair of sandals or flip-flops and show off those downright adorable feet.